LIVING

WITH

PARALYSIS

Real Answers You Need to Know, from Someone Living with Paralysis

JESSE GIFFORD

Copyright © 2021 Jesse Gifford

ISBN: 9798529492802 (Paperback)

First printing edition 2021. 5th Edition

DEDICATION

To my wife, family, friends, and most importantly my father, mother, and sister … I do not know where I would be today without your help, your support, and your unconditional love.

Contents

CHAPTER 1: WHO I AM

I am so glad you have chosen to read my book. I have overcome and learned a lot from my challenges over the years. I hope to accomplish three goals with this book. My first goal is to provide a road map for those newly injured or currently injured people who have a spinal cord injury (SCI) or other form of ailment that may cause paralysis. Second, I want to provide a resource for families, spouses, or caregivers, to better understand the needs of someone living with paralysis. Finally, I hope to give you answers to questions you may not know to ask or are maybe even a little embarrassed to ask.

My name is Jesse Gifford. I had an incomplete C5-6 spinal cord injury in 1997 when I was eighteen. After my injury, I was scared, lost, and had no idea what I would be able to do in the present and on into my future. I had to learn things the hard way. I did not always have resources or experienced people to show me the way. Doctors, nurses, therapists, and even caregivers do not always volunteer information, and in some cases, they just are not aware of essential information to give to someone living with paralysis. Even though I have lived with an SCI for many years, there are still things that come up that make me say to myself, *man, I wish I would have known about this earlier after my injury.* With that in mind, I want to provide you with the essential things I have learned over the years. I hope they will help you have an easier experience.

As I began to write this book, it was around the time of my twenty-third anniversary since my accident. My wife, Analisa, asked me if I ever think about that day, I had my injury. Of all days, it was Mother's Day 1997. I was eighteen. Me, my mother, grandmother, sister, aunt, and my cousin's girlfriend all got together for Mother's Day. We decided to go up into the woods near our favorite campground. This campground and general area were a favorite place that my entire family had gone to for as long as I could remember. We pretty much grew up running through these woods and swimming in the many creeks that flowed through the area. We had our favorite swimming holes that we would always go to, to swim. Today was no different. It was an unusually warm spring day. I loved the water, so naturally, I thought I needed to go swimming. The rest of my family was already down near our favorite swimming hole.

I quickly changed into my shorts at my truck and took off running through the woods. As I got close to the water, I was running at full stride. I pulled off my shirt, gave a yell of excitement, planted my foot at the edge of the water, and dove in. Everything went dark and became still. I was totally conscious but unable to move anything but my head and shoulders. I could not feel the frigid water surrounding me. I thought to myself, *my family is up the creek a ways and surely must have heard me yell. I just have to hold my breath long enough for them to get to me.* For about a minute, I held my breath as sensations and consciousness slowly faded away.

I began to see a light but was unsure of what was happening to me. I opened my eyes slightly to a flood of light. I then tried taking a shallow breath to see if there was air or water. Thankfully, it was air. I quickly exhaled and then inhaled as much fresh mountain air as possible. They had gotten to me and were able to turn me over but could not completely pull me out of the cold water. I lay partially submerged and unable to move for about an hour until help arrived. I was air-lifted to the nearest hospital, about twenty to thirty minutes away by air. My surgery took around five hours. They had to make a five-inch incision in the front of my neck, paralleling my esophagus, so they could gain access to my injured spinal cord. They created a fused bridge over the fractured area of my spinal cord.

My injury was an incomplete break, meaning my spinal cord was not completely severed. The break was located just about level to the top of my shoulders at the C5-6 level of my spinal cord. The first two weeks after my injury were spent in ICU. During that time, I fought to get off a ventilator. Shortly after the ventilator was removed, I developed pneumonia due to the ventilator or the frigid water or a combination of the two.

I spent another two and a half months in the hospital recovering and going through physical therapy. I was released just after my nineteenth birthday in August and went home to my amazing father, mother, and sister. Over the next year, I strived to get stronger and eventually could use about 50 percent of both arms. I could move my wrist up and down but had no finger movement at all. Everything else below mid-chest was paralyzed.

I accomplished my goal of getting strong enough to start college just about a year after my accident. Two years later, I began driving again on my own. Long story short, I graduated from college in 2004 with a computer science degree. I found a job a year later as a web and graphic designer for a publishing company. I worked until I got a pressure sore in 2010. That took me a year to recover. Unsure how my health would be, I had to go on Social Security disability. I eventually went back to work part time at an elementary school and also do freelance web design. I bought a house in 2013 and married Analisa in 2015. We have enjoyed a happy, healthy life ever since.

After all these years, I do not really think about my accident much anymore. The one thing that has always haunted me about my accident is *why and how did this happen to me?* I was an athlete who was co-captain of both the football and track teams in high school. I had been a lifeguard for several years at the YMCA. I knew where I was diving and that it was deep enough to dive into. The most bizarre thing is that I never hit anything in the water. I did not even hit the bottom. An SCI can happen to anyone at any time. It does not matter who you are, what kind of shape you are in, or how much money you are worth. I often thought about the how and why, but it never gave me answers or helped me in any way. I have always tried to look forward and focus on the things that need to be done and accomplish goals that I have set for myself, rather than dwell on what could have
been. I chalk it up to, *it must have just happened for a reason.* Maybe the reason is just to write this book to help you!

Parts of this book may be hard to read for someone new to SCI or paralysis. The positive thing you must keep in mind is that you are learning this information now. You are not always told the things you need to know. Being able to find the resources and knowing what is possible as early as you can will save you in numerous ways. I will also discuss important things you need to know about staying healthy. Looking back from my perspective now, a book like this would have been a positive game changer for me. So, through all my health issues, assistance issues, and personal issues that I have gone through, you will receive the benefit. You're welcome!

CHAPTER 2: IN THE BEGINNING

You take for granted how easily you can move. One day you stub your toe or get a cut on your finger, and you think your whole world is crashing down around you. Now, just think how you would feel if you lost feeling and movement in 50 percent, 70 percent or even 90 percent of your body. That stubbed toe is sounding pretty good about now, right?

It is hard to describe to someone what it is like to be paralyzed. It is a horrible feeling, thinking and knowing what you want to do, only to be stopped, trapped in a nonresponsive body that does not allow you to do the things you really want to do. You ask yourself; *how can I live like this? What kind of life can I have? How are people going to look at me?* This is just the start of the mountain of questions that haunt you after an SCI. It seems like your life is over and that you will never again find joy or happiness. You lie in your hospital bed numb, both physically and emotionally. The world as you knew it has been destroyed. Your present state has left you lost and confused. You try to deal with your injury, all the questions and the uncertainty that you now constantly think about, but it is too overwhelming. There still may be a chance you can recover. More likely though, you just hope to get some movement back. What do you do now?

I had all these feelings. I was in bad shape. I started out on a ventilator, feeding tube, oxygen, heart monitor, and whatever else they had me hooked up to, not to mention however they were controlling my bowel and bladder issues. I had a ventilator because the doctors were unsure if I had the muscle control to breathe on my own. The ventilator was eventually removed, and as it happened, I could breathe on my own just in time to develop pneumonia.

Pneumonia is beyond serious for someone with an SCI. We no longer have the necessary muscle control to effectively cough to clear our lungs of the liquid that builds up. So, if I did not drown the first time, I was now being given a second chance. Fortunately, I was able to recover and got off oxygen but not after I had lost close to forty pounds in just a few weeks. The feeding tube was also removed, thanks to the night nurse completely plugging it up using her own soda-and-hot-sauce concoction that was meant to clear the first obstruction. I had no appetite. With my feeding tube gone, I was left with two choices. Either, I would have to try and start eating on my own or I would have to get a feeding tube that would need to be surgically inserted into my stomach.

Through all that, the only movement I had was in my arms and that was even very limited. So, what did I do? Naturally, I cried and grieved; you have to. But you cannot stay in that mindset of sadness and depression. Your choices are rather simple at this point. You can choose to be that depressed person and think there is no hope. You can shut everyone out and shut yourself down until something eventually kills you. The other option is to get your life back. The only way things get better is if you make them better. You must change your mindset and fight for something. My something was my family.

My mindset was to get better for my mother, my father, and my sister. I did not want to ruin their lives or be a burden to them. This was also amplified with the occurrence of two events. First, in the beginning, my mother set one goal for me. Her goal for me was to become strong enough that I could put my arms around her and give her a proper hug. That is all she wanted from me. The second thing that motivated me was from my physical therapist who worked with me in the ICU. After only a couple days of working with me and seeing the movement I had, she said, "Oh, don't worry, you'll eventually even be able to drive on your own." She was probably able to see my jaw drop like she had said something offensive to me.

I wanted to say, *are you talking to me? Drive a car? Have you met me? I can't even pick my nose!*

So, now I had two goals: give my mother a hug and drive a car on my own. That is quite a spectrum of things to try to accomplish when you can barely move. How do I even do that, though? This is what I did. As already mentioned, you have to have the right mindset and improve your current situation for a reason. In addition, you need to start by setting small goals for yourself, so you can achieve small victories, which lead to bigger goals and bigger victories.

Initially, my blood pressure was low due to everything I had gone through and from lying in bed practically motionless. One of my first small goals was to work on improving my ability to sit up without blood pressure problems. Throughout each day, I would have someone raise the head of my bed up into a more sitting position so I could work on my stamina. That led to getting on a tilting table that could slowly tilt me up until I was in a standing position. Standing with the help of the tilt table led me to sitting up more and spending time in a wheelchair.

Another goal was to just start eating. After my feeding tube incident, I chose to start eating and forced myself to take one more drink or eat one more bite, even though it seemed revolting due to my lack of appetite. Setting this small goal along with having a former physical education teacher come in to visit me and forcing gummy bears into my mouth, led to eating as much junk food as I wanted so I could quickly gain back some weight. It was these small goals in the beginning that made it possible for me to go on to give my mother numerous hugs and get my second van because I drove the wheels off the first.

CHAPTER 3: SIDE EFFECTS

The human body is an amazing piece of junk! I always like saying that. It is funny, but it is so true. First, the human body is amazing. For example, the pure construction and process of being able to see is astonishing. According to the National Eye Institute, "When light hits the retina (a light-sensitive layer of tissue at the back of the eye), special cells called photoreceptors turn the light into electrical signals. These electrical signals travel from the retina through the optic nerve to the brain. Then the brain turns the signals into the images you see."

Alternatively, the human body is also a piece of junk. It is slow to heal, requires constant maintenance, is easily susceptible to infection and disease, and is vulnerable to heat and cold. If I created a computer program that was as unreliable and poorly designed as the human body, I'd probably be fired on the spot. The spinal cord and brain, which make up your central nervous system, fit into both these categories. They are both amazing and junk! The central nervous system goes beyond amazing. According to the Christopher & Dana Reeve Foundation, the central nervous system (CNS) controls most functions of the body and mind. It consists of two parts: the brain and the spinal cord. The brain is the center of our thoughts, the interpreter of our external environment, and the origin of control over body movement. Like a central computer, it interprets information from our eyes (sight), ears (sound), nose (smell), tongue (taste), and skin (touch), as well as from internal organs such as the stomach. The spinal cord is the highway for communication between the body and the brain.

For all its amazing capabilities, the central nervous system has one major flaw. If injured, the central nervous system, the most crucial and important system in your body, lacks the capability to regenerate and heal itself. "Some cells of the central nervous system are so specialized that they cannot divide and create new cells. As a result, recovery from a brain or spinal cord injury is much more difficult and sometimes, impossible."

So, now that I have a spinal cord injury, essentially injuring my central nervous system, what changes are going to occur in my body? Obviously, you are already aware of the first and biggest change-you cannot move! A lot of people are unaware of the secondary effects of living with a spinal cord injury and paralysis.

Muscle Spasms

We have all seen the movies or TV shows where the paralyzed guy stabs himself in the leg with a knife or fork to prove he has no feeling in his legs. I would not recommend stabbing yourself as a party trick at your next party. What the movies and TV do not show you are the aftereffects of the injury to your leg. Ordinarily, if you step on something sharp, that pain message travels up your leg, through the spinal cord, and to the brain. Essentially, the message tells your brain, *Brain, something bad is going on with your leg. What do we need to do?* The brain formulates a solution such as, *Take the foot off whatever is sharp.* The brain sends the message back down the spinal cord and to the leg, where the leg carries out the orders, all this being done in a split second.

What happens with an SCI when the communication is cut off between the body and brain due to the injured spinal cord? The body does a curious thing when there is pain below the site of your injury. Below your injury, you no longer feel pain, so the body reacts in the form of a muscle spasm. In basic terms, with an SCI, that pain message is still sent up your leg and up the spinal cord, where it tries to get to the brain for instructions. However, the message is stopped at the site of your injury because the path is severed or interrupted. The message is confused, returns to the site of pain, and initializes a muscle spasm to try to get away from whatever is causing the pain.

Muscle spasms generally consist of muscles tightening, fingers twitching, abdominal muscles vibrating, or your legs and feet thumping like you are trying to keep the beat to a very fast song. While living with an SCI, there is a fine line of whether muscle spasms can be an ally or an enemy. To explain, for the most part, muscle spasms are a good thing. The spasms give your otherwise motionless legs a little exercise. They are also a good alert of things happening in your body that you are otherwise unaware of. These spasms are also caused by minor irritations such as going over rough terrain or having your shoes tied or Velcroed too tight. Muscle spasms can also become the enemy by interfering with your quality of life. You might get to the point where your legs are spasming over every little bump or continuously without you being able to control the spasm.

A common medication to help control muscle spasms is called Baclofen. Baclofen is basically a chill pill for muscle spasms. It relaxes your muscles, so they are not as irritated. Baclofen comes in pill form or liquid form that is delivered using a Baclofen pump.

It is amazing how over time you can naturally adapt to most situations. Having lived with an SCI for twenty-three years now, at the time of writing this book, I have made my muscle spasms into an ally. I take six chewable Baclofen, spread out throughout my day (two when I wake up, one around 11a.m., one around 1p.m., one around 4 p.m. and one before I go to sleep). Six Baclofen throughout the day seems to be the sweet spot for me. My quality of life is good, yet I still experience muscle spasms, alerting me when something is wrong. Learn to listen to your body.

Over the years, I have learned to listen to my body through the different sensations that go along with muscle spasms. Yes, there are different sensations for the different types of pain that may cause problems throughout your body. Learning and knowing what those sensations are caused from is half the battle and something you must discover on your own. Exercise is also good for muscle spasms. Doing leg stretches, or range of motion, helps decrease muscle spasms. My extraordinary wife, Analisa, usually does different stretches with my legs in the morning to help decrease my stiffness and spasms before getting up.

Autonomic Dysreflexia

Autonomic dysreflexia is the big bad, bully cousin to muscle spasms. Autonomic dysreflexia is another way that your body is telling you something is wrong, only when this happens you better get relief now or things are going to get a whole lot worse. Autonomic dysreflexia can be life-threatening.

Here's <u>HealthLinkBC</u> to explain it better.

Autonomic dysreflexia is a syndrome in which there is a sudden onset of excessively high blood pressure. It is more common in people with spinal cord injuries that involve the thoracic nerves of the spine or above (T6 or above). Be prepared to call your spinal cord injury therapist, 911, or other emergency services if you or the person with the spinal cord injury (SCI) has the symptoms of autonomic dysreflexia. If you or a caregiver cannot treat it promptly and correctly, it may lead to seizures, stroke, and even death. Symptoms include:

- A pounding headache.
- A flushed face and/or red blotches on the skin above the level of spinal injury.
- Sweating above the level of spinal injury.
- Nasal stuffiness.
- Nausea.
- A slow heart rate (bradycardia).
- Goose bumps below the level of spinal injury.
- Cold, clammy skin below the level of spinal injury.

Milder symptoms of autonomic dysreflexia that I have experienced are flushed face, clammy skin, and nasal stuffiness. Although nasal stuffiness is not a 911 emergency, I have always found it to be the best, first indication I am getting too warm. Yes, sometimes the body is a piece of junk, but it still finds a way to give us a warning when something is wrong. Remember to listen to your body. I usually get these symptoms when I am up at the lake or just outside in general for an extended time when it is warm out. Another thing that adds to this pleasure is that I cannot sweat. My level of injury is high enough that the signal to start sweating does not reach my sweat glands. No sweating means no cooling down. Sweet, that must be great during a poker tournament! Not quite. You may look cool and calm on the outside, but on the inside, you are boiling. It is very easy to do.

I have found myself overheating numerous times. You are out in the warm sun for a while with your friends, your nose gets a little stuffy, and you start breathing a little harder, but you do not think that much about it, and you try to tough it out. It sneaks up on you, and you are warmer than you think. You finally go inside and have what I call a meltdown. It is much like drinking alcohol too fast. It tastes good, you are having fun, your friends are having fun; then you start to feel it a little, so you stop, but it is too late. The damage is done, and you are drunk.

With an SCI, getting over-heated is just as sneaky. Getting too overheated can cause more severe problems like heat-stroke and more severe symptoms of autonomic dysreflexia. If I get really overheated, I must have cool air blasting on me, while shirtless and chugging ice water. Still with all that, it takes me a couple hours to really cool down. When I finally cool down, I feel like a drained battery. You might say, all of that does not sound too life threatening though, Jesse. Oh wait, it gets better-I mean worse!

The worst symptom I have felt when experiencing autonomic dysreflexia is the pounding headache and sweating when I am not supposed to be able to sweat. This usually occurs if my bladder is not draining correctly and filling up or if I need to urgently defecate. This rarely happens though, if even once a year, but it is very serious. While your body senses something is wrong, your blood pressure begins to rise. It feels like the blood is shooting straight to the top of the inside of your skull and wants out. It is the worst and scariest pain I have ever felt.

I quickly must get out of my chair and lie down. We check and treat bowel or bladder issues. If those things seem to be fine, it is now time for a trip to the hospital. Luckily for me, it has never gone that far. We have always seemed to find the problem, knock on wood.

Catheters and Bladder Infections

Out of everything, people with an SCI most often say they want to get their bowel and bladder control back. At least I would. Unfortunately, with an SCI the loss of bowel and bladder control is common. The natural control occurs quite low on the spinal cord so there is a larger part of the spinal cord that could be damaged, blocking bowel and bladder signals. We now have another problem: How do you manage to urinate if you cannot tell when you need to? Also, what do you do if you cannot physically urinate? The answer is you will now need to use some sort of catheter. A catheter basically looks like a high-tech straw. The two types of urinary catheterization I have ever considered *are indwelling catheterization* and *clean intermittent catheterization.*

Indwelling catheterization means the catheter remains inside of you. Clean intermittent catheterization involves inserting and removing the catheter each time you need to urinate. Both types of catheterization come with their own pros and cons, and they both come with side effects. No matter which type of catheterization you use and how clean you are, you are still going to fight bladder infections.

Bladder infections are the side effect of having a foreign body inside of you and are common for people living with paralysis.

After I came home from the hospital, we used an intermittent catheter. That meant having a long, thin silicone straw inserted down through the opening of my penis and into my bladder every two to four hours. I hated it! I had to have help with it, it hurt, I had to monitor how much I drank, and I got an infection every other month. It did not work for me, especially with my goal of trying to go to college and eventually having a full-time job. Before starting college, I met with a urologist to go over all my options. I needed something that I would only need minimal assistance with and something that was not permanent, just in case a treatment was found, and I could regain function.

I decided on an indwelling catheter called a suprapubic catheter. To use this catheter, a small incision is made a couple inches below my belly button. This opening leads down to the bladder, which is also opened slightly. This entrance allows a flexible, straw-like silicone catheter to be inserted through my abdomen and into my bladder. The end of the catheter that is inside my bladder has a small balloon that inflates with water. Because of this balloon, the catheter remains in place and does not pull out of the bladder. On the end of the catheter that comes outside of the body there is a small port that allows the balloon to be inflated or deflated with the use of a small syringe of water. The catheter is then connected to another tube that runs down my leg and

into a small leg bag that can be emptied. Once the catheter is inserted into the bladder and the balloon is filled, urine can freely
flow from the bladder out through the catheter and down the leg to the leg bag.

I hated this catheter when I first had it put in. I hated the idea of having a tube coming out of my body and was always worried it would get pulled out. Those feelings went away over time. One positive to this was that I could drink all the water or liquid I wanted. I would not have to worry about how much I drank or when to empty my bladder like other catheter methods. Being able to drink more meant I had fewer bladder infections. I also needed very little help with it and eventually I could empty it on my own with an emptier, which I will discuss in the equipment section. Also, if ever they find a way to restore my function, the catheter can be taken out and the hole can be closed.

As I said, there are pros and cons to each type of catheterization. Being able to drink a lot of water and have fewer bladder infections is a positive for this type of catheterization. There are also a few cons that you should be aware of before going with an indwelling catheter. On rare occasions, the catheter can become plugged up due to biofilm (a gel-like substance) in the urine. This is usually more common when you have an infection or do not drink enough water. This is problematic because if your tube is blocked, there is no urine going out. If urine cannot go out, it builds up in your bladder and must go somewhere. At this point, if the bladder gets too full, it begins to spasm, like a hand squeezing a water balloon.

This pressure and spasming can cause one of three things to happen. First and best option is that there is enough pressure to push the blockage clear, and your tube will begin to flow normally again. Second and not so much fun is that the pressure pushes the urine out the natural way, and you end up wetting your pants. Third and most serious, the pressure could cause the urine to back up into your kidneys, causing kidney damage. If you think your catheter is plugged up, you may have to disconnect the catheter from the leg bag tube and use a large syringe full of sterile water to flush out the obstruction which is called *irrigating*. If that does not work, you would need to change the catheter.

Whether you are having trouble or not, you will need to change the catheter every two to four weeks normally. I found that changing my catheter every two and a half to three weeks works best for me. There are several steps you must follow when changing a suprapubic catheter. Always have a nurse or someone who has been trained on how to properly change the tube help you with the process. Be sure they get it far enough down into your bladder and that they inflate the catheter balloon. Even if you have someone help you, know the process yourself to make sure the person is doing the procedure correctly.

The one time that I had a problem with my tube was when a nurse in my urologist's office changed it. I was new to the procedure and was not watching. She had changed the tube successfully and sent me on my way. That night, while I was being turned in bed, the catheter popped out. The nurse had not filled up the catheter balloon with water. I also take oxybutynin or Toviaz to help prevent bladder spasms. Bladder spasms can still occur just from going over rough terrain or having an irritation to the bladder area.

With either type of catheterization, you are still going to get an infection. My usual symptoms that indicate I am getting an infection are dizziness and increased unusual muscle spasms. If it gets too bad all I do is just take a urine sample to the lab at my doctor's office for a urinalysis (UA). I like to have sterile urine cups at home so we can collect the urine and take it to the lab. After collection, the urine container must be kept cool, usually in an ice chest with ice or cool pack. Once that is done, you will need to deliver it to the lab within a half hour. It then usually takes two to three days for results to come back.

I remember the first bladder infection I had in the hospital after my accident. I had an unusual stabbing pain in my right shoulder. It was determined I had a bladder infection. I was unable to swallow large pills, so the nurse had to crush up an antibiotic called Cipro into some applesauce. With my first bite of applesauce, I almost gagged. Cipro has a very bitter, nasty taste, which was amplified by the taste of the applesauce. I have not had applesauce since! I have had Cipro, and although I have had many kinds of antibiotics to treat infections, Cipro, unfortunately, has been the worst and most common. Always follow your doctor's instructions.

Always take the usual full two-week prescription. Also, follow the dietary instructions of what to eat and not eat while on antibiotics. Antibiotics kill both good and bad bacteria. A probiotic can be helpful to restore good bacteria. Do not use antibiotics in excess or without instruction from your doctor because you could build up an immunity to it rendering it ineffective for when you really need it.

I try everything possible to prevent bladder infections. The first, best thing to do is drink lots of water throughout your day. There is a saying that goes, "The solution to pollution is dilution." Luckily, with the type of catheter I use, I can drink tons of water. In addition to lots of water, there are numerous claims and combinations of things that might help prevent infections. It has taken me about twenty-three years to find the combination that works best for me. First thing in the morning, I drink about a quarter of a cup of water mixed with a half a teaspoon (1,000 mg) of D-Mannose powder. D-Mannose is a natural sugar that, once in the bladder, acts like a magnet for attracting certain types of bad bacteria. It is recommended that you not eat or drink for an hour after taking D-Mannose, so that the bacteria have time to latch onto the D-Mannose. Once I drink it and go through my process of getting up, an hour has passed. When I am up and, in my chair, we irrigate my catheter to flush out my bladder. What that means is to disconnect the leg bag tube from my catheter and use a large syringe to shoot sterile water through my catheter and into my bladder. It is not just sterile water though.

My urologist suggested a combination of sterile water and a tiny bit of white vinegar for irrigating the catheter. A full description can be found at the Gillette Children's Specialty Healthcare site. Here is a suggestion for keeping things as sterile as possible. The syringe should come in a sterile package. Carefully open the packaging and remove the syringe. You can then pour the sterile water and vinegar into the sterile packaging. This makes a good container for taking the syringe and drawing water out of the container and into the syringe for irrigating. My urologist also recommended a certain kind of catheter. The catheter he recommended and the one I use is a silver Tube Latex Catheter 22FR 5CC LTX SILVR 12/CS. This silver-coated catheter supposedly reduces your chances of getting an infection. Once we irrigate the tube, I start drinking water, since it is also recommended to drink lots of water an hour after taking D-Mannose, to flush everything out. Three times a day (11 a.m., 3 p.m. and 8 p.m.), I take a prescription called Methenamine. Methenamine is an old type of antibiotic that is used to slow the growth of certain bacteria. Medline Plus gives the following description.

"Methenamine, an antibiotic, eliminates bacteria that cause urinary tract infections. It usually is used on a long-term basis to treat chronic infections and to prevent recurrence of infections." I also take two cranberry pills together that seem to help my fight.

There is one final thing that I have found that seems to help prevent my infections. Diet, specifically the things you eat and drink. I have noticed not only for my overall health but for my urinary health, reducing or cutting out red meat, sugar, and alcohol goes a long way to being healthy. Bacteria feed on sugar. Why go on living, though, if you cannot have these things? Eliminating these things is great for your body but terrible for your soul. I prefer to eat as healthily as I can and use these types of foods as rewards. I love a good burger, cookies, and cocktails, but I just try to limit them to once a week or special occasions. While doing all these things, my record for not having a bladder infection is a little over a year.

Bowel Care

The topic of bowel care is always the most awkward and embarrassing subject to talk about. It is also one of the most important subjects to talk about. To know as much as you can about this subject and find a routine that works best for you will save you from having accidents and will help you keep a healthy quality of life.

Being a quadriplegic with limited to no hand/finger dexterity, I found it easier to have assistance with my bowel program. After my accident, in the hospital we were taught to do my bowel-care program in bed using a suppository and bed pads. For years we did it this way, thinking that this was the only way to do it. Although we became efficient doing my program in bed, it was a little messy, time consuming, and occasionally I would have accidents throughout the next day due to insufficient elimination. Eventually, I hired a caregiver with lots of experience working with people who were paralyzed. He showed me a new way to do my bowel program that changed my life from the first night we started it. This process involves using a <u>Hoyer lift</u>. Hoyer lifts help those of us who are unable to transfer in and out of bed on our own. A Hoyer lift is a portable lift system that enables a caregiver to hydraulically lift a person from their wheelchair to a bed or even into a car. They not only help you transfer but provide a safer way for a caregiver to help so they do not hurt their back or anything else. Hoyer lifts are available in manual or electric.

For the person in the wheelchair, a giant strap with four arms is placed as far down behind their back as possible. The two lower arms go under and through a person's legs and connect to the lift. The other two arms go under each armpit and connect to the lift. Overall, the entire strap makes up a cradle. Using the lift, I am taken up and out of my chair and lowered onto my bed. After undressing, I turn on my left side and have a suppository inserted against the left wall of the inside of my bowel. I've found that an effective suppository to use is called a <u>Magic Bullet</u>. Next, we overlap a full-size bath towel and place it between my back and the Hoyer strap to prevent red marks or sores under my armpits or lower back. While I wait ten to fifteen minutes for the suppository to start working, a caregiver prepares my shower chair. The shower chair is basically a manual wheelchair with an opening in the bottom where I sit.

The caregiver puts in an 80/20 mixture of water and bleach into a good-size container, which slides on brackets underneath the hole of the shower chair. I am then hooked back up to the lift and raised up and positioned over the shower chair. I do not sit on the shower chair, though; I am only suspended above it. In this position, gravity helps things happen more quickly, cleanly, and efficiently. Once I am done, the container can be emptied into the toilet, and I can be lowered onto the shower chair to take a shower.

I have also been taught that it is good to get in a normal routine of doing your program on certain days and times throughout the week, so muscle memory can add to things going smoother. I usually do mine on Tuesday, Thursday, and Sunday nights. I used to do it in the mornings, but it took up a large part of the morning, and I often felt thrashed all day afterward. In addition to beginning to work, I could only do it in the evening. It is really for the best; I can get my program and shower done, which then helps me sleep.

As with everyone, diet is very important for helping things run smoothly. A healthy lifestyle filled with fruit, vegetables, and fiber has helped me. I also take a stool softener and magnesium-oxide for additional help along with a Gas-x to help dissolve trapped gas that is caused from sitting in a chair and not being upright.

Osteoporosis

One thing that is often overlooked is bone density and the risk of osteoporosis. Osteoporosis is the decrease of bone strength making the bones fragile and more susceptible to breaking. Sitting all the time, quadriplegics and paraplegics do not get the necessary weight bearing and exercise to our legs and hips that helps build and maintain strong bone density.

It was quite a while, even years maybe, before someone mentioned bone-density issues to me. I talked to my doctor, who referred me to an endocrinologist. I was given a bone-density scan, and it was found that I had the beginning of osteoporosis in my lower spine and both hip joints. I started on bone-density medication, and over the years, I have been on Fosamax and Actonel, which did not help too much. I have also taken Forteo, which helped quite a bit but comes with a health warning. Currently, I am on Reclast, an injection I have gotten once a year for the past two years. I no longer need this medication because supposedly it will stay and work in my system for several years. According to WebMD, "It works by slowing the breakdown of bone and keeping bones strong. It also helps to reduce the risk of broken bones (fractures)."

After my injection, the first year, my doctor and I noticed a dramatic decrease in loss of bone density. I no longer have low bone density in my lower spine; it is as hard as a rock. My hip joints are now stable but still weak. I get a bone-density scan once a year, and I will now be going to one every two years. I take calcium and vitamin D every day, usually after a meal, to help absorption. I do have a standing frame that allows me to be in a standing position. Being able to stand is good for my bones, but I am guilty of not using it a whole lot due to my schedule, and it is kind of a pain to get into.

Pressure Sores

Pressure sores or pressure ulcers are a constant concern to someone with limited movement. Pressure sores are most dangerous to quadriplegics because quadriplegics are unable to sense pain and cannot adjust their weight to sufficiently relieve pressure from sitting in one place for so long.

A pressure sore is formed by putting constant, prolonged pressure in one spot of the body without any relief. Sores are most common over boney, prominent areas of the body. For example, the tailbone is usually a prominent spot for a sore. The tailbone is boney and gets the most pressure while you are sitting. If you are sitting a long time on a firm surface and unable to adjust or lift yourself up, a pressure sore could occur. If you are not sitting on a soft enough surface, the bone and hard surface will create pressure, and the skin and flesh between the two will break down or become damaged due to lack of oxygen reaching that area. If you notice a red spot, here is a good trick to try. Press your finger gently in the center of the red spot and release. If the spot blanches or you can see a change of color, it is probably just a pimple. If the redness does not change, keep a close eye on it and pressure off it.

There are only two or three things I am afraid of, and one of them is a pressure sore. I think of pressure sores as the ninjas of SCI side effects. They form silently, and by the time you start showing signs you have got one, it is too late. Instead of showing signs something is wrong on the surface of your skin, sores first lack oxygen from pressure and begin to break down deep in your tissue near the bone. If that damage is caused, the flesh begins to die and travel upward until it reaches the surface in the form of a red-or worse, a white-spot. I have had three pressure sores over the years. One sore on the inside of my thigh was caused by a seat cushion. This sore took ten days in bed to heal. My second sore was on the heel of my left foot, caused by pressure from a shoe. With this sore, I had to keep it out of a shoe with no pressure and have weekly doctor visits for a couple of months for it to heal. Finally, my worst sore was just under my tailbone, which was caused by sliding down on a firm plane seat, while not being able to move back in my seat.

I spasmed and did not feel well until I got off the plane. Once off the plane, my symptoms seemed to get better and go away. The next two months, I had increased spasms that got bad. Toward the end of the second month, a red circle formed on my backside, just under my tailbone. Eventually, it grew and turned white in the center, much like a blister. It opened, and I had to have my first surgery to clean out the dead tissue so it could begin to heal. This sore took me a year in bed, two surgeries and weekly visits to the wound clinic to heal.

To combat pressure sores, I have an alternating air mattress (refer to the equipment section) on my bed, and my Roho Quadtro Select 9x12 adjustable seat cushion on my power chair. I also tip as far back as possible in my power chair. My chair has a power tilt feature that allows me to tip back up to about thirty-five degrees. I usually get close to a wall, so I can tip back and rest my head on the wall. It was recommended that I tip as far back as I can for twenty minutes every two hours. Since that bad sore, I have not had any more trouble with sores.

Medication/Vitamins

Medication is a necessary evil when you are paralyzed. The addition of vitamins and supplements to your diet can also increase your health and possibly even help you get off some medications.

In the morning, I drink about a quarter of a cup of water mixed with half a teaspoon (1,000 mg) of D-Mannose and two Baclofen. At 11 a.m. I take one Baclofen and a Methenamine. After lunch, I take a Baclofen, one stool softener (100 mg), two magnesium oxide (400 mg), two cranberry pills, and an Omega 3 fish oil pill. At 4 p.m. I take another Baclofen and a Methenamine. After dinner, I take one whole calcium (600 mg) and two vitamin D (2,000 iu each), one vitamin K2 (90mcg) for added bone and cardiovascular health, one magnesium oxide (400 mg), one zinc (50 mg), and another Omega 3 pill. When I go to bed, I take a Baclofen, Methenamine, and occasionally a vitamin C.

Doctors/Hospitals

Having the right doctors and getting yearly checkups are essential. There are at least two main doctors you should see on a regular/yearly basis. The first doctor you need is a primary-care medical doctor, not a nurse practitioner. This doctor is your general doctor and handles yearly physicals, lab work, and checkups, and is the first step to getting referred to specialists if needed. The second doctor you need is a urologist. A urologist provides care for your urinary tract. They can help manage catheterization, bladder infections, and maintain healthy kidney function.

When looking for a doctor, it is always a good idea to find one who has experience treating patients with spinal cord injuries. It is easier said than done, though.

I have a great doctor! Although, in the beginning, I do not think she had a lot of experience working with someone with a spinal cord injury. It is okay, though, because she listens to me, takes her time, and is understanding of my situation. Many doctors just do not listen, or they hurry through your appointment. I go to her for my yearly physical and for things as they come up. She is never hesitant to send me to a specialist to follow up on things or help if there's equipment that I need. Your primary-care doctor is also the best one to go to for a letter of medical necessity. If there is something specific that you need, you and your doctor will need to go over the requirements of this letter pertaining to the thing that you need. According to the Patients Rising website, a letter of medical necessity is a "LEGAL document wherein your doctor argues why you need a specific piece of equipment, medical treatment or test."

My second doctor is a urologist. I go to him for bladder and catheterization issues. He can test for bladder infections, which can also be done at your primary physician's lab. Through the urologist's office, I also have a renal ultrasound every year. This ultrasound is the same as they use to monitor pregnancies, only my bladder and kidneys get scanned for kidney stones, cancer, and potential catheter damage. Every two years, I also get a cystoscopy, which is where they take my catheter out and insert a camera down into the opening to observe my bladder.

My third doctor is an endocrinologist. I go to this doctor once a year to have a bone-density checkup. About a week before my appointment, I have a bone-density scan, which measures the increase or decrease of my bone strength.

Hospitals can be dangerous for people with disabilities. Always be sure if you need to go to the emergency room, it is for an actual emergency. People with disabilities are more susceptible to infections, which could potentially be more prolific in a hospital setting. If you are admitted, be sure to discuss things like medication needs and equipment needs with your doctor or nurse. Most specifically, ensure you will have some kind of air mattress or air bed for preventing pressure sores. Lastly, a good friend or family member to be an advocate or bodyguard is helpful. Hospital staff can be notorious for making mistakes, not understanding your needs, or just being unsympathetic. It is also nice having another person with you, especially if you feel rough and are unable to think clearly.

(For underlined web site links, visit www.gifdzn.net/books/)

CHAPTER 4: EQUIPMENT

There are a few pretty good pieces of information in this chapter for you, but there is only really one thing that is of vital importance when it comes to equipment. You need at least two of everything. What? You did not hear me? You need at least two of everything!

Your equipment will eventually break, stop working, or go flat. You always need a backup plan and a backup piece of equipment. That is sometimes easier said than done. In the beginning, you might not have or be able to afford two of everything. In some cases, you do not even realize you need two of some things. You will most likely accumulate things over time. If you do not have an extra of something, you should at least have a backup plan. Insurance would laugh in your face if you requested for them to pay for two power chairs at once. They will, however, pay for a second power chair after a certain number of years. You may start with a manual chair, then upgrade to a power chair, then eventually another power chair down the road. Never get rid of your equipment unless you know for sure you will not need it even for a backup.

There are numerous pieces of equipment out there that can make your life easier. Listing all the equipment that could help you could take up a whole book. Here are some pieces of equipment I have found most useful over the years.

Wheelchair/Power Chair

This is how I started. At first, I had a manual chair and wore pushing gloves to help get grip to push the chair. It is hard in the beginning when you are trying to find the right chair, getting it customized to fit you, and hassling with insurance. I found, whether it was for equipment or more physical therapy, it would be common for my insurance company to deny me the essential things I needed. I was told by a physical therapist once that insurance denying claims was kind of like their way of seeing how important it is to you. If you are denied and no longer pursue a claim, it is a way for the insurance to get out of paying for items. Before anything, make sure you and your therapist and/or doctor go over exactly what you need and why you need it. This is where the letter of medical necessity, mentioned earlier, comes in handy. If you do get denied, appeal the decision, and do not get discouraged. Unfortunately, sometimes it is all part of the game. Never stop trying!

I eventually got a power chair because I started college and needed to get around faster without help from someone. As I said, you always need a backup. The morning I started my first job after college, my power chair decided to stop working. There was a mad scramble to put together my manual chair, but luckily, nothing else went wrong other than being a little slow, maneuvering around the office. Selecting the right kind of chair is based on the individual's needs. The <u>Christopher</u>

<u>& Dana Reeve Foundation Wheelchair 101</u> website has a good guide to helping you choose the right chair.

My current chair is a Quickie P-222 SE. It is fast and narrow, so that I can easily fit into my van. On this chair I also have a tilting feature. As discussed earlier, the power tilt reclines me back far enough to relieve pressure on my hips and tail bone. This feature is for those of us who are unable to adequately push up to relieve pressure or easily reposition. There's also occasional maintenance that goes along with any wheelchair or power chair. Whenever something needs adjusting or fixing on my power chair, my wife and I would always have to look around the house to find the right tools or replacement parts. This was frustrating and annoying.

While walking through the store one day, we came across a small toolbox about the size of a shoebox. It had big compartments and little compartments, and we thought it would be perfect for storing all the extra pieces and parts to repair my power chair quickly. We call it our pit-crew emergency kit. We keep extra brackets, wires, wire crimpers, Allen wrenches, nuts and bolts, duct tape, zip ties, and whatever else we can fit inside of it. This is so handy to have because everything we need for my chair is in one place. When we go on vacation, we just grab the pit-crew kit and never have to worry that we forgot any essential tool or part to repair my chair. Also, with any wheelchair or power chair, always try to get solid wheels instead of inflatable. The last thing you need is a flat tire.

Seat Cushions

I have had several types of seat cushions over the years. Having the right seat cushion is crucial. Originally, my physical therapist and I tried to find the best type of cushion for my manual chair. We tried a cushion that was firm foam all around except the very back center, where my tailbone hits. This section had a large indentation of gel for my tailbone. Either the cushion or a spider bite created a small sore on the inside of my upper left leg. Taking no chances, I switched to an inflated seat cushion. I went on to use this for many years.

The seat cushion was great but came with one big problem. Although occurring rarely, after a time, the rubber inside would get worn due to movement and shearing, which created leaks, and the cushion would go flat. Imagine going down the freeway and having all four tires on your car go flat at the same time. This was serious! If the cushion went completely flat, my boney butt would be sitting on a hard plate, creating a pressure sore in minutes.

That brings us to my current type of cushion, which I have used for years. It is called a Roho Quadtro Select 9x12. This cushion is also an inflatable cushion, but it is separated into four quadrants or chambers. Like four tires on a car, there are chambers, the front right, front left, rear right, and rear left. Unlike my last cushion, now if I get a leak, only one "tire" goes down, and I have some time before I must switch cushions. This seat cushion comes with a valve in the front that you can release so all the air in the cushion is distributed, making -a customized fit for your behind. There are also more high-tech cushions out there, such as the <u>AquilaCorp Cushion</u>.

Air Mattress

This next piece of equipment has literally saved my butt over the years. It is called an <u>alternating air mattress</u> and is used to prevent bed sores. There is not much to it! It is basically an air mattress that goes over any bed and connects to a pump. We were never told about this after my injury. I went home and would have to be turned on my side every three to four hours during the night. We would put down eggshell foam and lots of other padding on my bed, and luckily, I never had a problem. I did press my luck over time, going longer without being turned, which was not wise.

In 2010, I got my bad pressure sore on my tailbone. After my first surgery, I had a second surgery performed by a plastic surgeon. He was the one who told me about this air mattress after all these years. He also gave me tips on how to prevent future sores. Since my powerchair had a reclining feature, I would need to tip as far back in my chair as possible for about twenty minutes every two hours. Using the alternating air mattress at night would also be beneficial. During the night, the pump alternates air pressure throughout the mattress. While I am sleeping, there's not constant pressure in one spot of my body. The pump is quiet too! We plug the pump into a wireless adapter which plugs into the wall and connects to my voice-controlled speaker that controls my smart home gadgets. Since then, I have been able to sleep on my back the entire night. As with any air-related piece of equipment, these pads will eventually get air leaks. You will need a patch kit handy or even an extra pad if possible.

Leg Bag Emptier

As promised in the catheter section, I need to reveal something that has given me extreme independence over the years. So, as I said previously, I can drink as much water as possible with my type of catheter. That is great, but another problem arises. How do I empty my leg bag on my own? This was a huge obstacle I needed to solve before I could go to college or work full time. I could not reach all the way down to the bottom of my leg bag by my ankle, pull my pant leg up, open the leg bag, and empty it into a toilet. I also could not rely on someone always being around to help me if I needed my bag emptied. We tried thinking of everything and finally found an electric leg bag emptier online. The emptier pushes up and secures into the opening of the leg bag and has two thin cords, one running to the battery on my chair for power and one running to a button attached to the side of my chair that I can push to empty the bag. I use a certain leg bag (LEG BAG DISP 28 OZ LARGE W/18" TUBING (1) LF #CT5174 found at Byram Healthcare). This leg bag is the only one I have found that allows me to use the emptier. When I am ready to empty the bag, I press the button, and the emptier releases the fluid in my bag until I stop pressing the button. Every night, we run warm water through the emptier. The opening of the emptier tends to get build up over time from sediment in the urine and can minimize the flow of fluid.

Leg Bag Strap

With a suprapubic catheter, you need a way to secure the tube from pulling or getting snagged on something. If not secured, the tube would be pulling, causing irritation and discomfort. Worst case, you do not want the tube to be pulled on hard enough that it might cause internal damage or get pulled out completely.

My solution to this problem was to use medical tape. For a long time, I used medical tape to secure my tube from pulling. As the tube came out of my body, I would form a two-to-three-inch arch in the tubing and tape the tube onto my skin. This worked fairly well, but over time, I ran into a couple of problems. One problem, it was always hard to find the right kind of tape. The tape needed to be soft but sticky. The tape needed to be sticky enough to stick to the tube but also needed to be sticky enough to stick to my skin but not overly sticky to cause irritation or redness to my skin. It was a balancing act most of the time. I found that a rubber foam type of tape worked the best. Another problem with taping the tube was that it would come loose or unstuck from my skin or tube from moisture or from moving around throughout the day.

After years of using tape, a caregiver who worked for me suggested I try a <u>tube strap</u>. I had never heard of or seen anything like that before. The strap Velcros around my thigh, midway between my hip and knee. The tube lays over the top of the strap, where there is another little strap that Velcros the tube in place so it cannot move around or be pulled.

Medical Supplies

You always seem to need medical supplies. Having a medical-supply company that you can rely on to have items in stock and is able to efficiently ship your supplies to you is a necessity.

The three companies I recommend are:

Liberator Medical (https://www.liberatormedical.com/)

Byram Healthcare (https://www.byramhealthcare.com/)

Allegro Medical (https://www.allegromedical.com)

Door Locks

Getting in and out of your house and being able to secure it are two separate challenges to someone with limited mobility. As you become more active and independent, you need a door you can open and close and be able to lock and unlock on your own.

My first problem with being able to open and close my door were actually two problems in one. First, the front door had a doorknob. Due to my lack of finger dexterity, I am unable to apply the necessary grip strength to turn a round doorknob. I required a handle-type door opener that I could easily slip my hand into and turn. My second problem in opening and closing a door came once the door was open. For example, if I were leaving the house, I could open the door and swing it open far enough where I could easily get out. Once I was across the threshold and outside the door, there was no way to reach back to the door handle and pull it closed. I needed a way to have the door retract back to me after opening, rather than having it remain open.

To solve this problem, I found a gadget called a Door Closer, that attaches to the top of the door. I used this for years, and it was great!

As soon as I opened the door and went out, the door swung back to me, allowing me to grab the handle and close it. Unfortunately, after years of use, the screws began to strip out, and the whole thing began to come apart. When we eventually had our doors replaced, we had spring hinges installed. These were ten times better, and I have not had a problem since.

Now that I could open and close the door, I was left with my last problem of how I would be able to lock the door. I had my door handle and could close the door, but now the locking system was the problem. Again, my lack of finger dexterity made it impossible to use keys. With some research, I found the solution to both problems. I found a keyless door lock with a lever handle. It has a handle for easy opening and a keypad to lock and unlock the door, essentially replacing the use of a key. They are expensive, but mine have paid for themselves over and over. The buttons are reasonably easy to push, you can set different codes for different people, and you can schedule them to lock and unlock.

Portable Ramps

Having a portable ramp often comes in handy. These ramps are great and come in various lengths. They also fold up nicely and are relatively light weight.

I always keep a four-foot fold-up ramp in the back of my van. I also have a six-foot ramp. It seems like whenever I go to someone's house, they have at least one step that I would not be able to get up and over if I did not have a ramp.

Smart Voice-Controlled Speakers

I hated voice-activated devices. After I came home from the hospital, our family got a computer. One of my mother's co-workers gave me an expensive voice-activated software system so I could dictate to the computer instead of typing everything. For late nineties technology, it was an impressive piece of software. Unfortunately, it took hours of training to get it to somewhat accurately, recognize my voice. Even then, it was slow and still did not recognize my voice thirty percent of the time.

Toward the mid to late 2000s I got a device that hooked onto the visor of my van, which connected wirelessly to my phone. With this device, I could call out and receive phone calls while driving using voice activation. It worked well about eighty percent of the time. The other twenty percent of the time, the device could not hear me, understand me, or would call the wrong person. By 2019, I was anti-voice activation. My wife found that Google and the Christopher & Dana Reeve Foundation were giving away free Google Mini devices for people with an SCI and their caregivers. She was all for it, but I was reluctant after my past experiences. I thought if it did not work, we could sell it, and I never like to turn down free stuff. We ordered two, and within a couple weeks we fell in love with them and even had an electrician come out to install wireless switches to make our home fully automated.

The voice activation on our device worked pretty much flawlessly. This voice-activated device and other similar brands can be game-changers for people with limited mobility. They were for me. With our system, I can turn the air mattress on my bed on and off, adjust lights, thermostat, and TV, just to name a few.

Universal Cuff

Early on during my rehabilitation, I was introduced to a universal hand cuff. This cuff was small and slipped over my fingers and wrapped around the top of my hand and underneath my palm. Since I have no movement in my fingers, I could not pick up or grasp a spoon or fork. Neither could I write with a pen or pencil. On the palm side of this cuff there is a slit where you can insert things like spoons or forks, so you can hold on to a utensil. I used this cuff with a spoon or a fork so I could eat. I could also push a pencil through it so I could type on a keyboard. I also used a pen to write with, and I use it to put a toothbrush in for brushing my teeth.

Although this cuff has helped me tremendously, they do stretch out and eventually must be replaced. Also, I began to dislike having to carry it around with me all the time. I always had to remember to bring it when going out to dinner, or worse, going to dinner and realizing I had forgotten it at home. For lack of better words, I found a new way and outgrew it.

Now I only use this cuff for brushing my teeth. I discovered a better way, where I no longer had to carry around a cuff. Using my fingers works even better. To explain, if I took a fork, I would start at the end of the handle. I would thread the fork handle under my pinky finger, along the top of my ring and middle finger and underneath my index finger. The index and pinky finger would secure the fork in place. I eat, type, and write this way! One negative thing is that whatever you use will cause pressure and redness on the top of the ring and middle finger. Occasionally re-adjust the object or take it out of your fingers every so often, and you will be fine.

Computer Accessibility

Computers are vital for many people living with a disability. Computers provide access to a wealth of information, the ability to communicate with the world, and in many cases provide employment to the disabled who work from home.

It can often be challenging to use a computer if you have certain disabilities. Fortunately, computers are extremely versatile in making accommodations.

The two most popular types of computers are the Apple (Mac) computer and Windows (PC) computer. Both the Mac and PC computers have accessibility features built into their operating system to accommodate people with disabilities.

The following links are accessibility features for each type of computer:

<u>Mac Accommodations</u>

<u>PC Accommodations</u>

(For underlined web site links, visit www.gifdzn.net/books/)

After I had used these accommodations for a while, even at the highest speed setting, using the keyboard keypad to move the mouse was too slow for me. I also needed a universal way to quickly be able to use any computer I came to. To explain, when I went to college, I would often be using many different computers in the computer lab throughout the day. Each time I left a computer and came to a different one, I would have to take time to set up the accessibility features on that computer before ever starting any work. It was a way that enabled me to use a computer, but over time I grew out of it.

I began practicing with the mouse and found that I could use the mouse and not have to rely on the accessibility features of the computer. I could place my hand flat on the mouse, and instead of using my fingers,

I used my knuckles to click the mouse buttons. Applying enough downward pressure and lots of practice, I got the feel for using a mouse. Instead of using my hand cuff, I kept a pencil through my fingers to be able to type quickly.

Fanny Pack

Fanny packs can be useful if you cannot reach, do not like, or need a backpack. Fanny packs allow you to have an easily accessible place to store a minimal number of essential items.

I have used a black fanny pack for years. I like getting black fanny packs, so they do not stand out. I keep it stuffed down on my right side between my leg and the side of my chair. I can securely put the straps around my armrest and clip it so nobody can grab it or run off with it. I recommend getting the packs with one large compartment and a smaller compartment. In the large compartment I keep my pills, snacks, dollar bills, license, credit cards, and important information such as my health insurance and AAA cards. In the smaller compartment, I keep my phone and credit card that I use most often. One negative aspect is that the zippers are small and hard to grab onto, so zipping the compartment closed is difficult. A way around this is to get key rings to put on the zipper tab. These are very handy for quickly and easily slipping your finger into. Also, I hook my key fob onto the key ring to quickly operate my van.

Water Pack

Having a water pack is a great way to stay hydrated and not have to get water every few minutes. A water pack easily hooks on to the back of your chair like a backpack. The drinking tube is long enough to come around and lie in your lap or off to your side.

I use this often when I am at work or on a road trip. The drinking tube is long enough to bring around and place between my fanny pack and the side of my chair. Having the water tube off to the side hides it but also provides easy access whenever I need a drink. These water packs come with cleaning tools, and they should be cleaned once or twice a week. I have two or three of them that I alternate, so I can be using one when the other is being cleaned or is drying. What is the rule of equipment? *Always have two of everything!*

Exercise

Having an exercise program and equipment to stay healthy and strong is crucial. Once I got out of the hospital after my accident, I used a manual wheelchair, which provided most of my exercise. When I began college and switched to using a power chair, I was no longer getting my pushing exercise. I had to create an exercise program to keep my strength and endurance up. In physical therapy, I used TheraBand's to work my arms. When I got home, I began using ankle weights Velcroed around my forearms. They were okay, but I would always need someone to help strap them on me. Eventually, I found dumbbells I could get my hand around that also had a strap that went above my hand to secure it, so I did not have to grip the dumbbell. The bad thing is, I have never been able to find those same dumbbells anywhere. For cardio workouts, I use a pedal bike that I place on top of a desk and can pedal with my hands. *(For underlined web site links, visit www.gifdzn.net/books/)*

CHAPTER 5: HELP THROUGH PEER SUPPORT

It was odd. For the longest time after my accident, I guess I was in denial that I had a disability, even though I could barely move on my own. I think I was in the mindset that I just had a temporary disability. I would recover soon. I can do this on my own. For those reasons, I never felt the need to talk to someone in a similar situation or seek out a support group. Although, in the hospital, I had people practically forced on me "Oh, you need to talk to someone! Oh, someone in a similar situation can help you!" Those things might have been true, but at the time, I just needed to figure things out on my own.

Eventually, I did become a peer mentor for people with new injuries. This was mainly because I could not say no to my physical therapist. She asked me if I would be willing to talk to people who were in a similar situation. The first person I began talking to was a man in his mid-to late twenties. He worked at a trucking company on the docks, where he was accidentally crushed by falling pallets full of merchandise. He not only had an SCI but multiple other broken bones and a black eye. He had a wife and kids. He was kind and determined to beat his injuries but at the same time a little scared about how his new injury would affect his family and what the future would be like for him. We enjoyed talking together, and I quickly formed a bond with him. I remember being in his room one day, and he told me to go over to the window. He was excited to show me the boat he had gotten, parked down in the parking lot. He not only had his family but now a new boat to inspire him to get better.

One day as I came in for physical therapy, I was told he passed away. I was just stunned and horrified. I did not think that I wanted to go on mentoring people. Being reminded that I did provide help and hope, I continued mentoring, and I eventually met people I am still friends with today. I am glad I continued mentoring. It is a good feeling to think that I might have contributed a little to their success in overcoming paralysis. It also shows me where I was and how much I have overcome to get my life back.

It is also important for your loved ones or caregivers to have support. My wife, Analisa, has been a longtime follower of the "Wives and Girlfriends of Spinal Cord Injury (WAGS of SCI)" discussion group on Facebook and Instagram. She finds it helpful to read about what other women are doing, how they do things, and what they are going through. She also likes helping give support to the other women in the group. I also follow groups such as the Oregon Spinal Cord Injury Connection.

We all deal with things in our own way. There is never shame in asking for help, especially when it comes to a life-altering subject like paralysis. If you are lost, have questions, or just want to talk to someone, there are numerous sites and resources out there.

My two favorites are:

<u>Spinal Cord Peer Support USA</u>

<u>Spinal Cord Injury USA Group</u>

(For underlined web site links, visit www.gifdzn.net/books/)

The Christopher & Dana Reeve Foundation <u>support page</u> is also a good resource. This page allows you to submit questions, request peer mentors, call and talk to someone, and provides resources, information, and advice for servicemen and -women living with paralysis.

(For underlined web site links, visit www.gifdzn.net/books/)

CHAPTER 6: HELPFUL SERVICES

After an injury, your first resource will probably be your hospital caseworker. This person can assist you with getting paperwork started for Social Security and health insurance, as well as inform you about other related resources.

The <u>Christopher & Dana Reeve Foundation</u> is another great resource for information. The <u>Paralysis Resource Guide</u> is a one-stop handbook to help people with paralysis and their families or caregivers navigate the world of paralysis. Other chapters cover topics that help one live successfully with paralysis, including travel, recreation and sports, home modification, signing up for federal benefits, and wheelchair selection. There are also chapters on resources for children living with paralysis, disabled veterans, and caregivers.

Benefits.gov

<u>Benefits.gov</u> is an "online resource to help you find federal benefits you may be eligible for in the United States." Their mission statement describes, "As the official benefits website of the U.S. government, our mission is to increase citizen access to benefit information, while reducing the expense and difficulty of interacting with the government." Their website has an easy-to-use <u>benefit finder</u> to quickly narrow down programs you may be eligible for.

Social Security

"<u>People with disabilities</u> may be able to qualify for one of two federal disability programs: Social Security Disability Insurance (SSDI) or Supplemental Security Income (SSI). *"*

The <u>Social Security Administration (https://www.ssa.gov/)</u> defines each program as follows:

1. Social Security Disability Insurance program pays benefits to you and certain members of your family if you are *"insured,"* meaning that you worked long enough and have paid Social Security taxes (<u>https://www.ssa.gov/benefits/disability/</u>).

2. Supplemental Security Income pays benefits based on financial need (<u>https://www.ssa.gov/ssi/</u>).

Social Security is most often the first, most important resource to turn to after sustaining a life-altering disability. Once qualified, you can begin receiving supplemental income, possible qualification for health insurance, and access to other benefits. You can even work while on Social Security. Social Security's, working while disabled <u>handbook</u>

is a good place to start for information.

After my accident, I qualified to be on SSI because I had a job for the previous two years before my accident. Once I began working, my benefits went away because I was earning too much money. Years later, I had to stop working and go on SSDI because of my pressure sore. I eventually recovered and could go back to work, but it was helpful having income while injured and unemployed.

Although the monthly cash benefits usually are not that substantial, it is still better than nothing. When you work, whether you are on SSI or SSDI, there are rules you must follow. Each program has its own different rules about things you can own, how much you can have in savings, and how much you can earn per month. One way to get around the *savings* regulations is with what is called an ABLE account. Oregonablesavings.com describes an ABLE account by saying, "After the Stephen Beck Jr. Achieving a Better Life Experience (ABLE) Act was passed by Congress in December of 2014, people with eligible disabilities could finally save for their everyday needs, invest in a tax-free account, and prepare for the future without losing their state or federal benefits." Look up your state's ABLE website for more information, and always know the rules, whether you are on SSI or SSDI. Even though these programs are helpful, it is still best to strive to improve yourself, so you do not have to be on them, which is sometimes easier said than done when you are living with a disability.

Department of Human Services (DHS)

Once you qualify for SSI or SSDI, you become eligible to receive help from the Department of Human Services, Seniors and People with Disabilities Program. DHS can provide several helpful services such as food assistance, employment resources, and help to provide for caregiving. Contact a local DHS office to learn more about the programs they can offer.

Vocational Rehabilitation (VR)

The National Rehabilitation Information Center describes Vocational Rehabilitation as "made up of a series of services that are designed to facilitate the entrance into or return to work by people with disabilities or by people who have recently acquired an injury or disability. Some of these services include vocational assessment and evaluation, training, upgrading of general skills, refresher courses, on-the-job training, career counseling, employment searches, and consulting with potential or existing employers for job accommodations and modification. These services may also vary depending on the needs of the individual." According to the brainline.org website, there are three ways you can qualify for VR services. "To become eligible for Vocational Rehabilitation services you must (1) have a physical, mental, emotional, or learning disability that is a real barrier to you getting a job, (2) need Vocational Rehabilitation services to prepare you to get, keep, or regain employment, and (3) be able to benefit from the services that will assist you to get and keep the job or benefit from independent living. If you receive Supplemental Security Income (SSI) and/or Social Security Disability Insurance (SSDI) you are eligible."

After my injury, my biggest goals were to go to college and be able to drive on my own. I did not want to be a burden on my family, and I wanted as much independence as possible. I was ready with my goals in mind. I had a physical disability that created a barrier for getting a job that met the first requirement for getting financial help from VR.

To fulfill the second and third requirements for needing services, I needed to meet with a VR counselor. I first met with a VR counselor when I was nineteen years old. The first thing he said to me was, "We don't help pay for your own vehicle, and we don't help pay for a sex-change operation." Um okay!

The counselor and I first had to create a formal plan for what career I wanted to pursue and how I would go about achieving it, along with the benefits it might offer. Creating a detailed plan of what I wanted to accomplish, how I wanted to accomplish it, and how long it would potentially take to accomplish were all things that needed to be finalized before receiving benefits.

Americans with Disabilities Act

The <u>ADA Network</u> states, The Americans with Disabilities Act (ADA) became law in 1990. The ADA is a civil rights law that prohibits discrimination against individuals with disabilities in all areas of public life, including jobs, schools, transportation, and all public and private places that are open to the general public. The purpose of the law is to make sure that people with disabilities have the same rights and opportunities as everyone else. (https://adata.org/) If you have <u>ADA related questions,</u> (https://adata.org/technical-assistance) the ADA Network provides information, guidance, and training about the Americans with Disabilities Act. For further information, visit <u>ADA.gov.</u>

(For underlined web site links, visit www.gifdzn.net/books/)

CHAPTER 7: CAREGIVERS

Finding a caregiver is not always an easy task. DHS is a good resource that can possibly help you financially afford a caregiver. They can also provide resources to help you find a caregiver. You could also hire a caregiving agency that will provide caregivers to you, or you can post ads on your own to attract caregivers.

The hardest thing about the caregiver process is finding someone reliable and trustworthy. I was lucky to have my mother as a caregiver after my accident. When the time came to have someone else help me, I wanted to go through a caregiving agency or post ads myself to hire a caregiver.

My first experience with hiring a caregiver began with posting ads. I eventually formed the usual four-step process of posting an ad, responding to those who have responded to my ad, setting up an interview, and lastly hiring the best person.

When posting an ad, I tried to keep it short and simple:
I am looking for an experienced and dependable (Full/Part) time caregiver for a fun, active (Your Age) year old (Male/Female)

quadriplegic. Hourly wages of ($$/hr.) with approximately (Number of Hours) hours a week, (Number of Days) days a week preferably on (Days of Week) in the (Morning, Afternoon, Evening). Duties will include (List all Duties). (Male/Female) is preferred but not mandatory. Nice private home in (City). Call and leave a message with your phone number and the best time to call you back. Thanks!

Once you start getting calls from interested applicants, call them back and find out three things. During the callback, find out a little about their experience, why they want the job, and schedule a time and place to meet for an interview. I try to meet potential caregivers at a coffee shop or somewhere outside so you can talk discretely. Meeting them at a coffee shop, for example, is a neutral location, so you are not inviting a bunch of strangers over to your home.

During an interview, start by reviewing their qualifications and reasons why they applied for the job. Next, you will want to explain the details of the job. More specifically, be totally honest about your requirements of the job, specific duties, days, and times that the person will be needed. Be ready to ask them a lot of questions. Do you have experience with the things I need? Are you looking for a long-term or short-term job? What is your schedule like? Are you flexible for emergencies, weekends, etc.? When can you start? Do you have a provider number?

A provider number tells you they have gone through DHS training and have been through a background check. If they do not have a provider number, they can go through the requirements to obtain one from DHS. Also, asking for and calling references is good too.

Lastly, you need to decide on the person you would like to hire. If you decide on someone, do not throw away the contact information of the other applicants, in case your first choice does not work out. Once you decide on someone and offer them the job, invite them to your place to show them the working conditions. Explain all duties again, the work schedule, and that work may be on a trial basis to make sure you are comfortable with each other.

Working with an agency can be less stressful than trying to find someone on your own. There are several advantages when using a caregiving agency. First, the agencies' caregivers have already gone through a background check and have proven experience in the job duties you might require. Second, agencies can often provide a backup person in case the first person has to take time off or is unable to show up to work. Lastly, agencies usually send numerous people over for you to meet and interview, so you can find the person who makes you feel the most comfortable. One negative that I have found when using agencies is that agencies have a lot of turnover, so you may not have the same people for very long.

Having your spouse help you is another option. Initially, I did not want to have my wife do any of my caregiving. Sometimes it is inevitable though; somewhere along the line, they will have to know how to help you, and if they are doing it enough to get paid, that is even better. I have an amazing wife! It was her choice to start helping me part time, not that I need a lot, but she can still work full time at her day job and do her own things as well. Unfortunately, not all states <u>support payments to a spouse</u> .

(For underlined web site links, visit www.gifdzn.net/books/)

CHAPTER 8: DRIVING

Wanting to drive is an excellent and achievable goal. Nowadays, the technology that is out there enables a lot of people with a high level of paralysis the ability to drive on their own. Although driving gives you great independence and is a worthy goal, going through the process of getting a vehicle, adapting it, and being able to drive can be lengthy. In most cases, the process may take up to a year.

The first thing you should do on your own or through VR is to have a driving evaluation done by a <u>Certified Driving Rehabilitation Specialist (CDRS).</u> The CDRS will suggest the type of vehicle you will need, evaluate your mobility and strength, and make recommendations on the type of hand controls and equipment you may require. If you go through vocational rehabilitation and driving is part of your plan, they should cover the cost of both meeting with a CDRS and for any adaptive equipment the vehicle will need. The VR counselor can also help you find a CDRS, although they should have one who works with them regularly. When you are ready to find a vehicle, your VR counselor can also suggest some local businesses that specialize in wheelchair vans.

There are also numerous businesses you can find with a quick Internet search.

An Internet search for wheelchair vans, mobility services, or mobility and accessibility equipment will result in finding sites like accessiblevans.com. Two companies I have worked with are abilitycenter.com and rjmobilityservice.com. The next biggest obstacle when wanting to drive is just being able to afford the vehicle. Remember VR's first rule? Vocational rehabilitation will not help pay for a vehicle, but they will help pay for the adaptive equipment.   Finding a vehicle and affording it is often tricky. Ideally, you want to find a vehicle that has the lowest number of miles and already has a ramp or lift installed. Depending on the miles and year of the vehicle, the price could be anywhere from $10,000 to $80,000.

If you are unable to pay for a vehicle, there are some resources out there that might be able to help with the expenses.

Here are a few sites to check out:

BraunAbility National Grants

BraunAbility State Grants

The Mobility Resource

Mobility Works

(For underlined web site links, visit www.gifdzn.net/books/)

The first time I was evaluated to see what type of equipment I might need, I had to travel to the University of Washington, and I live in Southern Oregon. This was the first time I traveled after my injury. VR should be covering your expenses, the evaluation, travel, hotel, and food. It was always a fight with my vocational rehabilitation counselor to get things paid, even though I was entitled to these benefits. He always tried to cut corners instead of being an ally in my fight to accomplish my goals. For example, instead of taking a direct flight to Washington, he tried to get me to take a train. From where I live, I would have to be driven an hour and a half to the train station, catch the train, travel to Washington, making several train swaps along the way, then travel from the train station to my destination, all to save a little money. He had no clue how hard it is to travel with a severe disability. I put my foot down, or rather my wheel down, and told him that would be unacceptable and why. Do not let your counselor take the easy way out. They are there to help you, not provide another obstacle for you. I know this does not sound too appealing, and that's part of the reason why I have written this book. These are the types of obstacles I have had to learn from and hope you can avoid. You are going to run into bad apples like this, but you just need to know your rights, and if all else fails, ask for the manager.

I was fortunate that my amazing parents were eventually able to buy me a reasonably priced used 1997 Dodge Caravan. The van had a lowered floor and a ramp that unfolded from out of the side door. For adaptive equipment, I needed reduced-effort braking, a steering tri-pin, hand controls for the gas and brake, and a computer system that would allow me to use things like blinkers and wipers. I also needed a lockdown system that would secure my power chair into place when I got behind the steering wheel.

I also needed a parking placard or permit. If you think you will need to use a disabled parking space when parking in parking lots, you will need a disabled parking placard/permit to display in your front window or a license plate that clearly marks that you have a disability. To obtain a permit, you will have to apply for the permit. Check with your state DMV to find out what is required to apply for your permit. Usually, you will be given a two-part form to complete. The first part of the form will be information about yourself. The second part of the form will need to be taken to your primary physician. Your physician will need to fill out the rest of the form. They will need to state that you do have a qualifying disability and need accessible parking. After the form is completed, return it to the DMV to get your permit.

Once my vehicle was complete, we were able to take it home. It took me a lot of practice and fine tuning to get used to the hand controls and basic driving. I found that wearing <u>wheelchair push gloves</u> while driving helped me. At first, my mother or father would take me out to a large parking lot so I could drive around without hitting anything. It was much like being a teenager again, learning to drive for the first time. When my father went with me, he was fine, but my mother would always hold on tight to her passenger armrest and the side of her seat. Having someone with a high level of paralysis drive her around for some reason made her a little nervous.

I eventually graduated to driving country roads, then finally around town. The first time I drove on my own, I was not scared; I was just very nervous. The whole time I was going down the road, I kept thinking, *this is crazy! How should I be allowed to drive on my own? What if something happens? What if I have a problem? What if...What if?* I did fine, though, and I have had a perfect driving record, knock on wood for the past twenty-plus years.

My wife and I bought my second van on our own. The process went smoother with VR the second time. The person we worked with was understanding, knew what she was doing, and was my ally instead of an obstacle. Both times of going through the driving process took at least a year.

(For underlined web site links, visit www.gifdzn.net/books/)

CHAPTER 9: EDUCATION & FINDING A JOB

In a global economy where the most valuable skill you can sell is your knowledge, a good education is no longer just a pathway to opportunity it is a prerequisite.

– President Barack Obama

Finding a job is hard enough. Finding a job and having a disability is even more challenging. Having every possible advantage when returning to the workforce only increases your chances of landing the job you want. If it is just reading a book, passing an exam, obtaining a license in a particular field, or getting a two- or four-year degree, anything you can do to further your education will only benefit you and reduce your challenges in life.

College

If your goal is to go onto college, you may be a little intimidated about where to begin or how you would even navigate college life. After creating your plan with VR, you will need to gather more information, both for yourself and your plan. The first place to start is the campus resource office or better, the disability-services office of the college you would like to attend. Every college should have a disability- services department in some form. They can help guide you through everything you need to know about starting the college process, making classrooms accessible, getting priority registration, and can help with things like taking notes or providing extra time on exams. On campus, disability-services can also answer questions about medical services and dorm accommodations.

I started at a community college, then transferred to Southern Oregon University, where I received a Bachelor of Science degree in computer science. I knew I wanted to go to college. Starting out, though, I was intimidated, had lots of questions, and did not even really know if it would be possible to keep up with schedules and homework. I had good experiences with disability-services at both the community college and the university.

Beginning at the community college, disability-services showed me around campus and answered all my questions. I was left with a feeling that even with a disability, it would be possible to continue my education. Starting out, there were three things I needed from the on-campus disability-services. First, by having a disability, I qualified for priority registration. Priority registration means you can be one of the first students to register for the classes. Second, the desks in the classrooms were not accessible. In each of my classrooms, a table was placed so that I would have a work area. Third, disability services provided an assistant who could take notes for me and help me between classes. It's a win-win! The assistant helps me, and in return they get paid for their work through the college.

I remember my first assistant. She was nice, a little older than me, and had two energetic young boys. She would help me do little things like get my lunch out of my backpack and rotate my books so I could be ready for my next class. She would help me and at the same time try to keep her two Tasmanian devil boys out of trouble. It did not work! One day, while she was distracted with helping me, one of the boys went over to the front entrance door and pulled the fire alarm. The entire college evacuated out onto the streets.

By the time I made it to the university, I only needed a few accommodations. I was more nervous though. The community college I went to was like a glorified high school, but now I was at a university. Again, on-campus disability-services reassured me that this next step would be possible. I met the director of disability-services and remember her showing me where my classes would be around campus. We would become friends, and eventually she gave me a job overseeing and updating all disability-services web pages for the university. We are still friends today.

As for accommodations, I no longer needed a note-taker, since I could do it on my own with my trusty pen through my fingers. I still took advantage of priority registration, but now I only really needed two types of accommodations. I needed the classroom relocated if the original location of the room was inaccessible, and I needed extended time on tests, since I wrote and typed slower.

Government Jobs

The USA.gov Jobs and Education for People with Disabilities page is great for someone looking for information about getting a federal job. According to USA.gov, there are three advantages of government jobs for people with disabilities: "The federal government has job openings nationwide in many different fields, uses a Schedule A, an optional, non-competitive hiring process that is faster and easier than the competitive hiring process, and provides reasonable accommodations to qualified employees."

Basically, to apply, you and your doctor will need to fill out a Schedule A Letter, which is proof that you do have a disability. You must have your doctor or qualifying service agency fill this letter out for you. When applying for a federal job, you must submit this letter and be qualified for the job for which you are applying. Here's where you can find the Schedule A Sample Letter and Schedule A Guide.

Finding a Job

There are jobs out there for everyone. Having a job gives you a sense of purpose and pride. Getting to Friday, knowing you put in a hard week, and receiving that paycheck is a rewarding experience. The following are resources you can use to help start your employment journey.

If you qualify for Social Security and need a good resource or some coaching, here are two programs that can be extremely helpful. The first is the Social Security Administration's Ticket to Work Program (https://choosework.ssa.gov/index.html), which helps with "Access to Employment Support Services for Social Security Disability Beneficiaries Who Want to Work." The second is called Employ Reward Solutions (https://employreward.com/). The ERS's mission is to "coach and assist beneficiaries with finding employment and providing resources for housing, transportation and more."

A tool you can use to gain an advantage for getting a job is called the Work Opportunity Tax Credit. The IRS describes this as a "Federal tax credit available to employers for hiring individuals from certain targeted groups who have consistently faced significant barriers to employment."

Whether you go to college first or just start working, the job-hunting process is the same. There are numerous resources and job-search sites out there for disabled people who are looking for a job. Some helpful sites I've used in the past are:

1. <u>Abilityjobs.com</u>
2. <u>Social Security Opportunities for Individuals with Disabilities</u>
3. <u>FlexJobs</u>

(For underlined web site links, visit www.gifdzn.net/books/)

I applied for many jobs and went on many interviews before getting my first job as a graphic designer at a publishing company. Through this, I got comfortable talking to potential employers about my disability.

Here is the process I usually use for getting a job outside of the home:

1. Once you have found a job you are interested in, look over the hours you will have to work, benefits, and wages it offers.
2. Do some research. Find out if it is a company you want to work for, where they are located, and how much driving time it would take to get to the job.
3. When you are ready to apply for the job, customize your resumé and cover letter to reflect the qualifications of that job. Make both documents highlight your best assets and accomplishments. Neither one of the documents should have anything about your disability, but do not leave out any achievements, such as disability organizations

you have worked for or any recognition you have earned for working with people with disabilities.

4. Submit your resumé and cover letter and officially apply for the job and be ready for a phone call. Be ready to answer a few questions about your qualifications. Know something about the business, and have a few questions of your own to ask.

5. After you have agreed on a time and date for the interview, the very last thing you want to do is ask about accessibility. I always found this to be a good time to mention that I have a disability and to find out if I can even make it into their place of business. I never wait until the day of the interview, show up, not have things accessible, and surprise the employer that I use a wheelchair. The very last thing I say in the phone conversation is, "I also use a wheelchair, Is your office accessible?" This makes the employer somewhat aware of your situation and allows you and them to make accommodations if needed.

6. Once you are in the interview, be confident, emphasize your strengths, and if it comes up, give examples of how you have overcome your weaknesses and obstacles. I also like to have five or six questions for them. I usually print my questions out so I can hand them the paper to read and answer. At the same time, you can also have another printed document explaining the <u>Work Opportunity Tax Credit</u>.

7. If you are successful and get the job, you can then go over reasonable accommodations you may need to perform your job. Vocational rehabilitation is also a good resource for you if you have accessibility issues. Also, for accommodation questions, the <u>Job Accommodation Network</u> (<u>https://askjan.org/</u>) is a great free resource.

Always make sure to thoroughly look over and understand what an employer is offering before accepting a job. To explain, always know how the employer's benefits, like health insurance, will interfere or help with your current insurance and services. Also, be aware of how much money you will be making with a new job. Any supplemental income or services you are receiving could be affected by your salary.

(For underlined web site links, visit www.gifdzn.net/books/)

CHAPTER 10: TRAVEL

America the Beautiful Access Pass

According to the USGS (https://store.usgs.gov/access-pass), the America the Beautiful Access Pass is a "free, lifetime pass available to US citizens or permanent residents of the United States that have been medically determined to have a permanent disability (does not have to be a 100 percent disability) that provides admittance to more than 2,000 recreation sites managed by five Federal agencies."

I have had my pass for over fifteen years. If you are into the outdoors, it is well worth your time to get this card. I use mine mostly to get into national parks for free. For more information and instructions on how to get an Access Pass, go to the USGS (https://store.usgs.gov/access-pass) to find out more.

Flying

I do not really fly much, but when I do, I can only tolerate about two hours of flight time. I hate flying, but I love Las Vegas! I guess it is a necessary evil; fortunately, Vegas is only about an hour and a half flight from where I live.

There are six steps I go through when flying. The six-step process is packing, checking in, priority boarding, flight, disembarking, and luggage pickup.

Packing:

Packing is often difficult. If you are like me, you must pack not only your clothes but also your supplies, tools, and equipment. There is so much stuff you must remember to take that my wife and I needed to make the process easier somehow. We created a checklist. A travel checklist is a great way to make sure you take all your necessities. I usually keep my list on my phone in my Notes app. When we are ready to pack, I just take out my list, find each item on the list, and go.

Checking in:

When you arrive at the airport and get to the counter to check your bags, inform the counter agent that you have medical supplies in your luggage. If you let them know there are medical supplies in your luggage, they are required to allow the luggage to exceed the weight limit at no additional charge. Also, while they are tagging all your luggage, be sure to get a tag for your power chair or wheelchair. Once you are through the check-in, proceed to security. Security will pair you with an agent who is the same sex as you, male to male, female to female. This agent will escort you through security and have you sit off to the side, out of the way of people being screened. Here the agent will do a physical pat-down of you and your chair. Before they begin, they usually ask if you have certain items or if there is anything they need to know before beginning. Inform them of any leg bag, tubing, or miscellaneous things that may be underneath your clothes.

Priority Boarding:

Once you are through security, you will need to locate your flight gate. When you arrive at your gate, go to the gate counter, and inform the agent of your situation. You will need to inform the agent that you will need two things. First, you will have to ask for priority boarding. Priority boarding means you need to get on first because you need more time and/or help getting into your seat, unless it is a large plane, and you have the option of staying in your chair. Second, you might have to request an aisle chair and extra help with transferring into your seat.

When the plane arrives and they call for priority boarding, go to the front counter or near the terminal door. You will be escorted down the terminal walkway and must park right outside the entrance to the plane. Here you transfer into an aisle chair, which is a small chair on wheels that is just wide enough to fit down the aisle of the plane. It's terrible! Before transferring into the chair, we bring along a square foam pad to place on the seat of the aisle chair, since it is a hard surface. Did I mention it's terrible? I also need help transferring, which consists of one person lifting under my knees and one person behind me lifting under my armpits. Once I am awkwardly sitting in the aisle chair, they strap me down with several seatbelts, and into the plane we go. Transferring onto the plane seat is just the opposite of transferring into the aisle chair.

Your power chair or wheelchair will be taken and stored underneath the plane. Before they take it, I tell them not to tip it over on its side and to leave it upright. Also, be sure to have someone take stuff off your chair that might break or be torn off like the arm rests, footrests, joysticks, etc. Especially, take your seat cushion and maybe even your back rest off your chair. After my pressure sore incident, we began taking my seat cushion off and putting it on the seat of the plane.

Flight:

Once you are sitting in your seat, try to position yourself the best you can or have someone help you move back if you are too far down in the seat. Just get comfortable! To pass the time, Analisa and I usually have a two-player game on our phone that we like to play.

Disembarking the Plane:

When the plane lands, we are no longer priority. We are the last to get off the plane, dead last. We must wait for everyone to get off before they wheel the aisle chair in for me. We now go through the reverse order we went through of getting on the plane and hope my power chair is intact and still operating. (There have been times it has not been.)

Luggage Pickup:

By the time everyone has gotten off the plane, I am just getting back in my chair and headed to the luggage pickup. The whole process easily takes forty-five minutes. When we get to the pickup area, it is not uncommon that all our luggage is in the unclaimed luggage office. If you do not see your luggage in the pick-up carousel, do not worry; just check this unclaimed luggage office first. Fortunately, I make Vegas worth going through all this torture!

Lodging

It is always frustrating when you are on vacation and arrive at your destination, only to discover that your room is not accessible. When booking a room or vacation getaway, you must be meticulous about making sure it meets your accommodation needs. If you have a place in mind, envision arriving at your destination, and think of questions you would like to ask before booking. Does the establishment have accessible parking? Do they have a ramp and accessible entrance? Is the doorway to my room and bathroom wide enough for my wheelchair? If you rent a house, is the bedroom located on the first floor? Is the shower accessible? How high is the bed? These are just a few questions you might want to think about. You might even want to call and go over all your concerns with a manager before booking, rather than hoping for the best.

I have several tips that may help you on your next trip. First, be aware that if you get online, there are different types of accessible rooms. A resort or hotel might list a room as accessible, but that does not mean it has all the things that make it wheelchair accessible. If a room is listed as accessible, it usually only means that the basics are accessible like a lowered peephole, lowered closet rods, and maybe a shower chair or bench (available on request). Always read the amenities or accessible features section about the room to be sure it accommodates all your needs.

An accessible room usually does not have an opening under the bed for a lift to roll under for those people who might need to use a lift to get into bed. An accessible room also usually has a lip or step up and over into the shower, which does not accommodate a wheelchair. If you need to use a shower chair to roll into the shower, you need to look specifically for a room that is listed as an Accessible Roll-in Shower room. If you find one listed as a roll-in shower, make sure it says *roll-in shower* in the accessible features description and title. Even then, try to find a picture of the shower to prove it is accessible. When you check in and get to your room, check the shower to make sure it is accessible. I have gone through all this before and still was given a bathroom that you had to step into the shower instead of having a roll-in shower. Second thing you might want to investigate is if the resort or hotel offers accessible equipment. Some places offer shower chairs or lifts that you can use.

For more information about booking accessible rooms, flying, cruises, and all things travel, a great resource is https://wheelchairtravel.org/

CHAPTER 11: RECREATION

Everyone needs a hobby or physical activity. You have to find something that interests you, something that takes your mind off things and something that you can look forward to. When you have a disability, it is sometimes hard to find something you are interested in and able to do. You still might be able to do the things you once loved, but now you might have to do them differently. Alternatively, you still might be able to do the things that you once loved to do before your disability, but now you just cannot do them the same or as well, which takes the enjoyment out of it.

It is like being able to eat your favorite food but not being able to taste it. Does it still bring you the same enjoyment if you cannot taste it? Finally, you might just not be able to do those things you once loved. That is when you need to find new things that interest you. You have to start trying new ways of doing things, finding hidden talents, discovering things you did not know you would like, and having new experiences.

Growing up, I was always an athlete and an outdoorsman. After my accident, a lot of the things that I loved doing, I could no longer do.

There were still things I could do that I once enjoyed, but now I was not as good at doing them. I did not get the same enjoyment out of them any longer.

I was a different person now and needed to find different things that would give me joy. We got our first computer after I came home from the hospital. I had never been interested in computers and never really cared to take the time to sit down and play with one. Now I had one and obviously had the time to learn how to use it.

I started playing with the computer, which led to going on the Internet, which led to researching how to build web pages, using code, and soon how to design to make it all look good. I discovered I had a talent and interest in both coding and design, which grew into going to college and eventually getting a job in that field.

As for recreation, I always loved the water and the outdoors. Kenny, a friend of our family, offered to take my dad and me out on the lake in his nineteen-foot powerboat. We accepted but were not sure how I would do on a boat or if I could even get into the boat. To get me into the boat, Kenny not only lifted me in but also put me in the captain's chair so I could drive. Driving the boat was a little awkward and intimidating at first, but I quickly caught on and found that it was something fun I could do.

After that experience, we began looking for a boat to buy. It happened that a family friend was selling his nineteen-foot powerboat. He ended up giving us a good deal. It was great and something fun I could do with friends and family. I still had to be lifted in and out of the boat. Being lifted was not ideal for me and especially not for the person lifting me. My family and I began brainstorming about what we could do to make the process easier on everyone. My mother thought of the idea to put in a hydraulic lift system. Taking the idea, with the help of a few friends with engineering skills, we created a system that worked great.

To explain, we made a ramp that went from the dock and connected to a platform just big enough for my powerchair, which was in the back center of the boat. I would go from the dock, up the ramp, and onto this platform. The platform was on a manual scissor-jack hydraulic lift system. Once I was on the platform, the release valve could be turned, and the platform was lowered into the boat. We had a similar system underneath the captain's chair. So, I would be lowered into the boat, the captain's chair would be pumped up, even with my powerchair, so I could transfer across. When I was in the captain's chair, I would then be lowered into position behind the steering wheel, and my powerchair could be pumped back up and taken out of the boat. When I was ready to get out, we would just do everything in reverse order.

It was so great to be out on the water and having fun with family and friends. It made me feel almost normal again. Our lift system even made it into a couple of disability magazines. It is important you find something you are interested in that also gives you enjoyment. Do not use your disability as an excuse not to try things. You might find things that change your life that you would have never known about otherwise.

Gaming and Virtual Reality

For many, gaming is a good way to bond with people, make new friends, and escape your reality for a while. The reality is that there will be quite a few things that you once loved to be competitive at, but you will just not be able to physically do them anymore. It is important that you try new things and find something that excites you. I have never been a good spectator. I have always loved to be competitive. Of course, after my injury, I was not able to compete in a lot of the things I once loved. I did find things I could still be competitive with, but it was frustrating because I knew I could do them fifty times better if I did not have a disability. The inverse was also true. There were games I became better at after my disability. My family had always been into playing shuffleboard. After my injury, I found that I had more feel and concentration for the game. I now have a shuffleboard table at home and have shuffleboard tournaments several times a year. I also found I enjoy hosting murder mystery parties and playing video games.

Video games have gotten very popular, and the technology has advanced quickly. For disabled gamers, though, the technology has not advanced quite as fast. Many of the controls for gaming systems, understandably, are designed for the abled masses. These controls are often unusable or frustrating for disabled gamers. I love racing. After my accident, my dad or cousin and I would always play racing simulator games against each other on two computers. It took a while for me to get good. I would use a steering wheel and steer it with my left hand. I would then have the computer keyboard angled along the right side of the steering wheel. With my right hand, I could press one button for the gas and another button for the brake.

Most games now allow you to program which button you want to use for each game function. This is great, but if the controller is not very accommodating, it really does not matter. In the last few years (of writing this book), Microsoft has made the greatest advancements to help the disabled gaming community with their release of the <u>Xbox Adaptive Controller</u>

The controller acts as a central hub. Adaptive controllers like <u>joysticks</u> and <u>larger buttons</u> can be plugged into the main controller. The advantage is that you can control any function within a game, with a controller that works best for you.

Gaming is a great way to form bonds and find new friends. Gaming also gives you a sense of equality and helps to take your mind off your disability. Be open to trying new things. If something does not quite work for you the first time, do not give up. Think outside the box and try to figure out a way that it will work for you.

Virtual reality headsets are the next level of gaming. You still use controllers, but it's not always a problem since many of the games only require you to press one or two buttons. You can also play many of the games just by holding the left and right controllers and moving them around. Since I'm unable to grasp a controller, the controllers have attached Velcro straps that you can put your fingers through that hold your hand in place so there is no way to drop either controller even in strenuous games. Virtual reality is not limited just to games. It also allows you to virtually explore the world, watch Youtube videos, browse the Internet, hang out in virtual social environments, and so much more. It often makes you feel like you don't have a disability.

Many Other Things

Of course, these are just a few examples of the ways I have fun. There are many other things out there that allow a wheelchair user to be active. I have one friend who has the same level of injury as I, and he is an active paraglider. Another friend is a skier. Just doing a keyword search for *wheelchair sports* returns numerous pages of possible sports you would be able to play in a wheelchair. The website <u>Disability Friendly</u> lists the twenty-one best wheelchair sports you need to know. You are only limited by the disabilities you place on yourself.

(For underlined web site links, visit www.gifdzn.net/books/)

CHAPTER 12: RELATIONSHIPS

After an SCI, you question a lot of things. The one thing you will most likely question is if it will ever be possible for you to be in a relationship. Who would ever be attracted to me now? How will it be possible for someone to see me and not my chair? What will this do to my current relationship? That is just the start of the questions you might be asking. Although the answers might seem bleak in the beginning of your disability, if it is something you want, and you work for it, it is something you can get.

Luckily, I was not in a relationship at the time of my accident. I say that because I had enough stuff to worry about (like surviving) and needed to focus on me and what I needed to do to get better. I did eventually get better and got to a point in my life where I felt that I could start dating and have relationships. Yes, no matter how much you think it is not possible, someone out there will find you attractive if you keep trying…sometimes you do not even have to try! I had doubts about myself in the beginning too, but come on, I'm irresistible! Finding the right one for me took a while, though. You may want it, but it is tough out there, especially with a disability. Do not make your disability your excuse, though. Yes, you will be dumped, stood up, cheated on, and all the fun stuff that goes along with dating, but disability or not, that is everyone's story.

I prefer to think that having a disability helped me. How? The women who did not give me a chance were not worth having in my life anyhow. The relationships I did have that did not work were missing something and needed to end. This finally brings me to finding the right one that I eventually married.

Analisa and I met online and talked for quite a while before going on a date in 2013. At this point, I was a master planner! I hated wondering what to do during a date or asking each other, "Well, what do you want to do?" "I don't know, what do you want to do?" I had our first date all planned out, except for a small speed bump halfway through the date. Seriously, it was an actual speed bump! We met at her favorite Mexican restaurant, where I surprised her by waiting outside with flowers. Told you I was irresistible! We had dinner and I then drove us to get ice cream for starters. It was dark by then, and we parked in the last accessible spot in the row along the strip mall where the ice-cream shop was located. Of course, there was no curb cutout to go right up into the ice-cream shop. In the dimly lit parking lot, I had to parallel the entire row of shops before I could get to the cutout at the very end of the parking lot.

I have a fast power chair. Being a guy, I thought I would show off my speed, so I gunned it while she waited for me to come around. Just as I got up to full speed, I hit an unpainted speed bump and probably looked like a crash-test dummy. Once I came down out of the air and came to a stop, my keys were on the ground, I slid halfway down in my chair, my leg was having a muscle spasm, and my foot was about to come off the footrest. On top of all that, I was too far down in the chair to move back on my own, and the car I landed behind was about to back out and leave. Luckily, they saw me, got out, handed me my keys, and ask if I was all right. Playing it cool, I said I was fine, thanked them, and cautiously made my way down to the cutout and back to the ice-cream shop.

I got to where Analisa was waiting and had to stop to see if I could move back in my chair. I was too far down in the chair, and even after several failed attempts I could not get back on my own. Analisa volunteered to help me, and I knew this relationship would be different. I proposed to her in 2014 (with the help of Hall of Fame running back Emmitt Smith) and we were married in 2015. Analisa is the kindest, most innocent, loving, joyful, and trustworthy person I have ever met. We are happy together, have gone on tons of adventures, and our only regret is not meeting sooner.

(For underlined web site links, visit www.gifdzn.net/books/)

CHAPTER 13: SEXUALITY & PARENTING

It is a misconception that if you are paralyzed you cannot have sex or even have children. Yes, it is not quite the same, but with a little education, imagination, and medical intervention, both are possible.

For men, the natural ability to get an erection and ejaculate is controlled from the lower portion of the spinal cord in the sacral area (S2-S4). Once paralysis occurs and communication along the spinal cord is interrupted, the natural male function is disrupted and no longer functions correctly, if at all. It is still possible to get erections with stimulation, but they are most often random and non-sustainable. Men basically have three options for achieving an erection: with injections, a pump, or medication.

How to Solve Erectile Dysfunction

When I was newly injured, I remember a urologist talking to me about storing sperm. A procedure can be done to extract sperm, then store it for a future time when you would like to use it. As for getting an erection, getting an injection every time ... um, ouch, no thanks! A pump always seemed weird and awkward, so I have relied on medication.

It is never fun talking to your urologist about these things, but it was made even worse the first time I talked to my urologist about getting medication. I was taken back to one of the patient rooms, where the nurse did the usual blood pressure check and standard questions about my medications and overall health. She finished and just before she left the room she said, "The doctor will be right in, in a few minutes."

I had it all planned out about what I wanted to say. I thought it would be easy! I would take two seconds to ask him, and he would take two seconds to write out a prescription. It would be done, and I would be out the door. An hour later, I was a nervous wreck and still waiting for him. I had repeated a hundred times what I was going to ask the doctor and was just about ready to leave, when he came flying through the door. The whole appointment was a blur until the very end, when I asked his thoughts about a suitable medication.

He was totally understandable, but my insurance did not cover such medications. Instead, he said, "Oh, wait, I'll just get you some samples!" He burst through the door to the little nurse's station right outside. Of course, every attractive nurse in the office was there doing paperwork. "Has anyone seen Patty?" he asked. Patty was the physician's assistant and just happened to be a longtime family friend. Just great! Luckily, she was busy somewhere else as he began to rummage through the cabinets, enlisting everyone else's help in locating the samples. He finally found the packets of medication, and like a kid in a candy store, he started stuffing a paper bag full of these samples. He returned, plopping the bag down on my lap as I tried to get out unnoticed and as fast as humanly possible.

I eventually began taking Sildenafil. The Mayo Clinic recommends, "Adults up to 65 years of age—50 milligrams (mg) as a single dose no more than once a day, 1 hour before sexual intercourse." The recommended dosage on the container says to take three to five pills, but for me I take one to two and it always seems to do the trick.

Having Children

According to Spinalcord.com, "Only around 10 percent of men with spinal cord injuries are able to conceive naturally (if they use erection medication). For the rest who cannot, they are turning to the best two options available penile vibrators and the surgical extraction of semen (which is used to inseminate an egg and then implanted in a female) known as in vitro fertilization (IVF)" (Accessed June 10, 2021). Unfortunately, both options are usually not covered by insurance. The cheaper of the two options is the penile vibrator, which starts at a couple hundred dollars and can be used at home. Of course, always consult your doctor with questions you may have, and be aware of possible health risks. The Johns Hopkins Medicine website details a penile vibrator as "A specially designed mechanical vibrator that is placed at the base of the glans penis and is set at a certain frequency and amplitude. Men with an intact ejaculatory reflex arc, which is dependent on the level of spinal cord injury, are able to experience reflex ejaculation.". Penile vibrators can be found on sites like Fertility Healthcare Inc. (https://medicalvibrator.com/) along with other supplies to aid in sexual dysfunction.

CHAPTER 14: LIFE IN GENERAL

How do you feel after reading this book? I threw a lot at you! You may be feeling overwhelmed, scared, or confused, wondering how you are going to do all of this. Don't worry, I have been there too! My hope, though, is that this book at least gave you one or two a-ha moments, and you discovered or learned something that will help you overcome challenges in your life. I also wanted this book to give you hope and clarity that there are better ways of doing things and that there's assistance out there for when you need extra help.

An SCI is not the end of your life; it is just a different path. It is not the path you planned on or wanted, but now you must make it the best path you can possibly make it. Along the way, you might even discover a life you never knew could exist.

The things I have learned and achieved now, I would not even have thought possible twenty-three years ago, lying motionless in that hospital bed. I have discovered talents and interest in design, programming, and finance that I never knew I had. I accomplished my goals of giving my mother not one hug but numerous hugs over the years and not only driving a car but a ski boat too. I graduated from a university, held jobs, bought a house, got married, and reached my main goal of being extraordinarily normal. I could not have done it without my determination, wife, friends, and most importantly, my father, mother, and sister.

<u>Important:</u>

Please, leave a **REVIEW ON AMAZON!!!**

For the full web site link to all <u>**UNDERLINED**</u> words visit, http://www.gifdzn.net/books/. Click on the Living with Paralysis book and click, ***BOOK LINKS*** at the top.

Finally, a portion of the profits from this book go to the <u>Christopher & Dana Reeve Foundation</u>, so please share this with someone you think would need it.

Thank you,

Jesse

ABOUT THE AUTHOR

Jesse Gifford was an exceptional athlete, member of the National Honor Society in high school, preparing to attend college, and had just been sworn into the Army National Guard when he sustained a spinal cord injury paralyzing over half his body at age 18. Now after living as a C5-6 quadriplegic for over 25 years, he's overcome extraordinary obstacles to achieve a Bachelor of Science in Computer Science, home ownership, employment, written two books, and has a wonderful marriage. He now strives to create the best life possible both physically and emotionally, as well as financially. His primary focus is to share with others, his secrets for overcoming both physical and financial challenges.

For more information and to see my other books, visit

www.gifdzn.net/books/

Copyright © 2021 Jesse Gifford